Hold Fast
A man's journey through grief, fatherhood, and the quiet war of PTSD.

P.J. Lyons

Hold Fast: A man's journey through grief, fatherhood, and the quiet war of PTSD.
© 2025 P. J. Lyons

All rights reserved. No part of this book may be reproduced, stored in a retrieval system, or transmitted in any form or by any means - electronic, mechanical, photocopying, recording, or otherwise - without prior written permission of the author, except in the case of brief quotations used in reviews, articles, or scholarly works.

This is a work of nonfiction. It reflects my life as I remember it, told as honestly as I can. Some names and identifying details have been changed to protect the privacy of individuals. Certain events have been compressed or adjusted for narrative flow, but the heart of the story - the truth of what was lived and felt - remains my own.

ISBN: 979-8-218-72139-8

Independently Published

First Edition: 2025
Printed in the United States of America

For my brother, who taught me to believe.
For my father, who taught me to carry it.
For my mother, who carried more than I ever knew.
For my sister, who loved me even when I disappeared.
For Lizzie, who never stopped fighting.
For my children—Rannon, Declan, Mairin, and Flynn—my reasons.
And for DC, who answered the call.

A NOTE TO THE READER

Hold Fast is a work of nonfiction that explores themes of grief, trauma, and post-traumatic stress disorder (PTSD) with unflinching honesty. It includes vivid depictions of Coast Guard and military operations, as well as candid reflections on suicidal ideation, emotional withdrawal, and the ripple effects of trauma on family life. If you are in a vulnerable state, or have a personal history with these issues, please proceed with care. Your well-being is what matters most.

If you need immediate support, you can reach the Suicide & Crisis Lifeline by calling or texting 988 in the US and Canada. If you are outside these regions, please contact your local emergency or mental health hotline for help.

CONTENTS

	XI
Prologue - The Call	XIII
1. When the Noise Stopped	1
2. Where It Really Started	15
3. Far From Perfect	25
4. The Four Corners of Me	35
5. Cracks in the Ice	45
6. Bleeding In	55
7. The Disappearing Act	65
8. She Stayed	71
9. Diagnosis	83
10. After the Storm	93

11. The Unsent Letters												103

You have to go out, but you don't have to come back.
Attributed to Patrick Etheridge, US Life-Saving Service station keeper.

PROLOGUE - THE CALL

The ship sat in its berth at Cape Canaveral, Florida, idling in a kind of quiet readiness. Lines coiled, diesel engine humming somewhere below. We were set to cast off any minute, another patrol, another day on the water.

Then the intercom crackled to life: "Petty Officer Lyons, phone call."

I froze. Nobody calls me when we're underway.

It didn't feel urgent, but it didn't feel right either. Just off. Like the air shifted and I hadn't caught up yet. I picked up the receiver.

It was my father.

"Pat . . . something's happened. Your brother . . ."

And then nothing.

He couldn't say the words. The silence on the other end said everything.

Then my sister's voice took over, shaky, wrecked, trying to hold me and crush me all at once.

"Jay's dead... Something happened during a race."

My knees gave out. I didn't speak. I didn't move. I dropped where I stood. A man in uniform, crumpled to the deck of a government ship, holding a phone like it might bring him back.

Chapter One
When the Noise Stopped

I didn't realize how loud my life had been until the silence hit me in Rockland, Maine.

I was eighteen. Fresh out of USCG boot camp. Lying on a stiff mattress in a room that smelled like mold and boredom. Government issue everything, white walls, plastic drawers, a desk no one wanted to sit at. I couldn't sleep. Not because I wasn't tired but because there was no noise.

I had grown up with a city soundtrack—sirens, traffic, muffled yelling from the street below. Even at night, Quincy breathed. But Rockland? Just cold silence and the occasional moan of wind off the harbor. The walls creaked like they were trying to speak, but they had forgotten how.

I'd lie there, eyes wide open, heart thudding like it didn't know what to do without background noise. The silence wasn't peaceful, it was oppressive. My thoughts got louder. They filled the space left by the sirens and shouts. Every regret. Every insecurity. Every *"what the fuck am I doing here?"*

That was the first time I felt truly alone. Not just physically but stripped of anything familiar.

Growing up, I never noticed the chaos because it was constant. My sister Paula and I would bicker over nothing. My parents moved like machinery—work, dinner, TV, sleep. It was clockwork. And Jay, my brother, Jay was a full orbit ahead of me. Eleven years older, already in motion, already someone. I was still figuring out how to lace up my skates when he was applying to colleges. Still whispering to our dog, Muffin, under the table while he was moving out of the house.

I was raised Irish Catholic in suburban Boston, and that came with its own quiet doctrine. You went to Mass. You wore the right clothes. You didn't make a scene. Emotions weren't forbidden, just . . . tightly managed. Grief belonged at funerals. Joy belonged at weddings. Anything in between got folded into the day's chores.

The men in my family weren't cold, they were steady. Reliable. My dad included. He didn't always say much, but you felt what mattered in the way he showed up. Love wasn't loud. It was built into routines. Shoveling the driveway before anyone asked. Fixing what broke without needing thanks. That was how care was communicated—through action, not conversation.

Still, I grew up learning that certain feelings didn't have a place. Sadness got swallowed. Vulnerability got redirected. You could laugh, you could yell, but you didn't say you were scared or lost. That wasn't our way. Not out of cruelty but because that's how they were taught, too.

And so, I learned to carry things quietly. To show up, hold steady, and figure the rest out later.

Muffin was our family mutt. Gray face, old soul. She'd shuffle under the table and rest her head on my lap while I sneak-fed her scraps. Mashed potatoes, pieces of chicken, crusts from grilled cheese. We had an unspoken deal: She took what I gave and never snitched.

One day, she wasn't there. I asked where she was. Dad said Jay lost her. Just like that. "Jay lost her." I held that against him for years.

Only later did I find out they had to put her down. Jay had taken the blame to protect me from the truth. That was his way; he'd shoulder it, so you didn't have to.

Even if you hated him for it. Especially if you hated him for it. That stuck with me.

Jay was already living in the Mods at Boston College by the time I was hitting puberty. Dad and I would visit on football Saturdays. The place was alive, with music thumping and students tailgating, red Solo cups in hand.

I remember the first time he handed me a soda and introduced me to his friends, saying, "This is my little brother." Just like that, I belonged. I walked taller that day. Watching him in that world was like watching a celebrity at home. He had it. Confidence. Charisma. Control. I wasn't jealous, I was studying.

We used to have this autographed Larry Bird poster in our room growing up. Jay got it somehow, probably through one of Dad's connections or some random hustle. It hung right above our shared dresser, Bird mid-layup, signature in silver ink sharpie. When Jay moved out, he let me keep it. No ceremony, no speech, just said, "It's yours now." I kept that thing for years, through every move, every shitty apartment. It made it all the way to North Carolina with me. Then one day, moving back to the Cape, it vanished, lost in the shuffle of boxes and cheap tape. I still think about that poster. Not because of what it was worth but because of what it meant. It was ours. His. Mine. A little piece of him that stayed behind. And now it's gone too.

One summer, we played a round of golf out on Nantucket, just the two of us, hacking through tall grass and pretending we had a clue. On one hole, I absolutely smoked a drive . . . first time ever, really, except I didn't yell "Fore."

I yelled "Jay!"

He turned, looked, and—*boom*—dropped like a cartoon character, no blood but stunned, holding his head while I sprinted over, already apologizing.

We laughed about it later, hard, but I never forgot the sound. The thud. The way I yelled his name instead of the warning.

It feels loaded now, in hindsight. Like I was trying to protect him too late.

The thing is, even when you try to follow someone's path exactly, you never walk it the same. Jay was discipline and stability. I was chaos wrapped in charm. He trained for triathlons. I trained for late nights and hard hits. He was measured. I was all instinct. But I still wanted to be him. Or, at least, the version of him I carried with me.

After college he moved west for work, and I went to visit him in California. He was living with Karen, his girlfriend, later his wife, and they had a parrot named Jake that hated everyone except Jay. Jake would scream, "Where's Jay?" whenever he left the room. It was absurd and hilarious and somehow perfect. Jay had built a life I didn't even know how to picture.

One afternoon he brought me to meet his friend Dave—DC. The three of us ended up driving out to Petaluma to see a Coast Guard ship tied up there. I didn't realize it then, but that trip would change everything for me.

Standing on that deck, listening to them talk, seeing the uniforms, the ship, feeling the sense of purpose in the salt air, it lit something in me. Until then, the Coast Guard had been just a word, a vague idea. That day it became real. Tangible. A path I could see myself on.

Looking back, I realize that was a pivot point. Jay and DC didn't just show me a ship, they opened up a doorway. And for whatever reason, I stepped through.

Years later, DC would die in a helicopter crash in Afghanistan. Another name added to the list of people I couldn't hold on to. Sometimes I think about that, how the men who helped set me on this path never lived long enough to see what it became for me. Another loss I carry.

The last time I saw Jay in person was at Falmouth Country Club in 2006. Just the two of us. It wasn't a big day, no milestone, no party. Just a casual round. I was about to move to North Carolina. He knew it was a big change for me, but neither of us treated it like a goodbye.

I told him it was my last tour. That after this, I was getting out.

He raised an eyebrow. "You sure?"

I remember laughing, brushing it off like I always did. But he had a way of reading through the cracks. He knew I wasn't sure. Not really.

I remember the way the sunlight hit the greens, the way we talked about everything and nothing. I remember how he lined up his putts like they mattered. I remember thinking I'd see him again soon.

And then I didn't.

Once I moved south, we'd have the occasional phone call. The last time we spoke, it was just a regular call. One of those check-ins that feels small until it isn't.

Jay had been training for a triathlon. Pushing hard like always. He told me he was feeling good, ready for race day. I remember teasing him.

I said, "Nobody ever got hurt sitting on the couch."

That was the last thing I said to him.

It wasn't meant as anything. Just a throwaway line. A joke. Something you say to push your big brother a little. But it sits with me now . . . deep in my chest.

Because then he was gone.

I've thought about that line a thousand times since. What I meant. What he heard. What I'd say now, if I could.

He was swimming the Cohasset triathlon. Fit. Focused. Doing everything right. And then, just gone. I was in Florida, on our way to begin migrant interdictions. I caught a flight home, numb the entire time. I looked out the plane window and felt like the sky was pressing down on me. Not sadness. Not even disbelief. Just pressure. Like something heavy was crawling into my chest and making itself at home.

Even being there, it didn't feel real. His death didn't land in one blow; it came in echoes. In the quiet. In the way my dad cried. In the way my mom said his name. In the way I stood still while everything around me moved.

I went back to work. Because that's what you do, right? You keep showing up. But something had changed. I didn't feel like a version of myself anymore. I felt like a placeholder. A body going through motions.

I used to think guilt was something dramatic. A courtroom confession or a deathbed whisper. But real guilt? It's quiet. It moves slow. It lives in the back of your throat and under your ribs. It shows up when you're brushing your teeth or driving to work or lying awake at 2:00 a.m. thinking, *why him? Why not me?*

I was the reckless one. The one who ignored signs. The one who carried weight I never spoke about. Jay was steady. Strong. Ready for more life. He ran. He trained. He ate right. He lived clean. I didn't. But here I am. Still breathing. Still standing. Still trying to figure out why.

I think the last time I knew who I was, really knew, was when I first came to the Cape.

I was living on base at Otis. Young, dumb, and full of some kind of hope. I had a Jeep Wrangler that leaked rainwater and had the infamous death wobble. And for a little while, Rannon was living there with me.

His mom had since left the CG, returned home to Nebraska, and joined the Navy. She was eventually deployed, and I was figuring out fatherhood on the fly.

Diapers, bottles, naps—I was twenty-two and guessing every step. But I loved having him with me. We'd drive around Cape Cod with the top off the Jeep, his car seat strapped in, music playing. People probably thought I was out of my mind. Maybe I was. But it was the first time in my life I felt like I was showing up for something that mattered.

We got a yellow lab and named her Husker for Rannon's Nebraska ties. She was wild and gentle all at once, just like him. That little family of three was everything to me.

Until one day I had to fly out to bring Rannon home, and when I got back, my dad had given Husker away. Just like that. I didn't even get a say. "It was too much," he said. "You're never home." I didn't argue. I just swallowed it. But it was another quiet grief. Another thing I didn't get to hold on to.

I didn't realize how much those years shaped me until later. The Otis years. The Jeep. The dog. Rannon's car seat in the back. My hands on the wheel. Even now I can see clearly that version of me before everything spun out. Before the silence came back for good.

This is where the story begins.

Not with one loss but with a lifetime of unspoken things. With a blueprint I was trying to follow and then had to bury. With a mutt under the table. With city sounds replaced by Coast Guard silence. With the question no one ever asked me out loud: *Who are you now?*

And the truth is, I didn't know.

The funeral was surreal. The air was heavy. Floral arrangements lined the altar like a maze of condolences. I could smell the lilies before I even made it through the door. The lighting was soft, but nothing could soften the punch of seeing his photo on a tripod at the front of the church, him grinning like he was still here.

There was no casket, no urn, just a memorial Mass at our local parish. I don't think I could've handled seeing those anyway. It was hard enough imagining it. I just stood there with my head down like I was waiting for permission to breathe.

Before I even made it to the house that morning, Lizzie was already there. Not just showing up, showing up right. She didn't bring flowers or a casserole. She brought bagels and toilet paper. It sounds ridiculous written out like that, but it was exactly what we needed. That's Lizzie. While everyone else was frozen in place or lost in the chaos of grief, she was scanning the house for what was missing and filling in the gaps without fanfare.

She moved through the kitchen like she'd lived there forever. Quiet. Steady. Present. Not asking what needed to be done, just doing it. It was one of those moments when you realize someone isn't just part of your life, they're built into it.

We weren't married yet. We were still figuring things out. But that morning, without a word, she made it clear she was in it. Not just for me but for the whole damn storm.

In the church, my mother sat in the front row, eyes swollen, hands gripping tissues like lifelines. She looked smaller than I'd ever seen her. Paula sat beside her, stoic but twitching. Every so often, she'd reach over and rub Mom's back, then clench her fists again. I don't remember walking; I remember floating. People kept saying things—"He was one of the good ones." "He loved you so much." "He'd be so proud." "You're just like him."—but their words were hitting a version of me I wasn't in.

Chris Haun was already there. He'd gotten to the house before I did. Held space with my parents before I could get there. That's who he is. He'd hugged me hard at the wake, didn't say a word. He didn't need to. Just his presence said, *I got you*.

I didn't cry there. I waited until the car ride home, after everything had quieted down. That's how I've always been. Public armor, private collapse. It's like my grief needs silence before it'll show up.

Even now, I sometimes forget that I watched it all happen, the fall, the funeral, the aftermath. I was there. I really was. But in my memory, it plays like a movie someone else told me about.

A short time after the funeral, I went back to work like nothing had happened. I stood watch. Ran drills. Laughed at dumb jokes in the galley. I kept my boots shined and my hair short and my grief shoved so far down I almost convinced myself it wasn't real. It felt like pretending to be human.

But grief doesn't respect your schedule. It shows up when you're brushing your teeth or folding laundry or walking past a photo you forgot was there. It's slow and rude and it doesn't knock.

Lizzie and I had only been together a little while, but she already knew the parts of me I usually kept hidden. One night I lay in bed and stared at the ceiling, not saying a word. She reached over and touched my hand. Just lightly. No questions. No pressure. Just presence.

She didn't ask me to talk. She just stayed.

And in that silence, different from the Rockland silence, not empty but full, I let myself breathe. Just for a second. Just enough to remember I was still alive.

I didn't cry. But I wanted to. And that was new.

Chapter Two
Where It Really Started

I used to think trauma had a shape. Something obvious. Violent. A car crash. A shooting. Something that leaves blood on the floor and sirens in your ears.

But mine?

Mine wasn't like that.

Mine was responsibility too early. Being the kid who stayed quiet so the house stayed calm. Mine was hearing, "You're fine," when I clearly wasn't.

The truth is, I'd been carrying weight long before the uniform. Some things you inherit before you understand what they are. I just didn't have the words back then, not for the pressure and definitely not for the fear.

That feeling of being expected to hold it together while no one else even admits something is broken has never really left.

When my brother died, something in me went silent. I collapsed, I cried, but I also went right back to work. Back to the mission. Back to pretending it didn't gut me.

Only a short week or so after the funeral, my bags where packed. I kissed Lizzie goodbye and caught a flight to Key West out of Boston. I hadn't even begun to grieve, there wasn't time.

I sat by the window, watching the sky shift, numb to all of it. I didn't cry. I didn't think. I just stared. Somewhere over the Carolinas, it hit me. I had no idea what the hell the world even held for me anymore. Whatever compass I had was gone.

When I landed, a small boat brought me out to meet the cutter. Business as usual. Right into migrant ops. No time to catch my breath. Shave chits, search patterns, and tired routines.

I was down in the Florida Keys, back in the middle of migrant interdictions. One life leaves, and I'm pulling another out of the water. One body gone, and I'm processing logbooks like I'm still whole.

The guys—my crew—were incredible. Quiet support. The kind that doesn't ask questions but makes sure you're fed and your rack is squared away. They didn't push, didn't probe. Just made space. That mattered more than they'll ever know.

I remember the day Jay died how fast they moved to get me home. Got me off the ship and on a plane before I could fully register what was happening. To this day, I'm not sure who paid for the flight. I just remember standing at the airport, stunned, waiting for something to feel real.

I remember this one interdiction, a group of twenty-five or so, sunburned, soaked, and half-conscious. But we'd seen worse. We processed them and handed out water and gray blankets. I was doing my usual rounds, just checking in with folks, when I sat down next to an older woman wrapped in a blanket. She looked sixty, maybe older. Worn, cracked skin, deep eyes.

I asked if she was okay.

She looked up and said, "Doce."

Twelve.

At first, I thought I'd misunderstood, but she smiled and said, again, "Doce." It was her twelfth attempt to cross.

We'd caught her every single time. And she kept trying.

That stuck with me in a way I still haven't been able to shake. That broke something open in my worldview. I'd grown up believing in systems, rules, laws, order. But she wasn't trying to break anything. She was trying to live. And she didn't look angry. Just tired. Resigned. Resilient.

That was the day I realized it doesn't matter how many times you get turned back if what you're leaving is worse than the risk of starting over.

The crew kept me moving. No one asked too many questions, but everyone looked out. That kind of support you'd expect in the military. Ryan and I used to smoke cigars on the fantail. He'd kept my humidor running while I was back home for the funeral, made sure the cigars didn't dry out. Said it was the least he could do.

Doc, Sara, Mike—they were solid. We didn't talk about feelings, not directly. But they made sure I had coffee, made sure my rack was squared away, made sure I knew I wasn't alone even when I felt like a fucking ghost.

I listened to Grateful Dead albums during night watches. Caught Sox games on the radio when I could. Anything to make it feel like I still existed in the world. Most nights, it didn't work.

I wasn't sleeping. Not really. I'd close my eyes and see him, Jay, laughing at me from the golf course or standing in our old bedroom or worse... not there at all, just the outline. A hole shaped like him. I'd snap awake in a sweat, chest tight, like I couldn't catch my breath.

I thought I was just tired. Burned out. Nothing a few beers and a weekend off wouldn't fix.

But the fuse was already lit.

I'd lose track of time. Find myself zoning out during briefings, staring through people instead of listening. The world around me got duller, like I was watching everything through a fogged-up mask. I wasn't angry, not at first. Just... gone. Disconnected.

I didn't talk about it. Not with anyone. Because, in my mind, grief wasn't something you aired out loud. It was something you carried. Quietly. Like a good man. Like a strong man.

But the silence didn't heal anything. It hardened it.

I didn't know it then, but I was already showing signs: emotional numbness, hypervigilance, survivor's guilt, the whole list.

But it wasn't some dramatic breakdown. It was slow. Creeping. Like rust in the seams.

I kept telling myself I was fine. And I kept showing up like I was. Until one day I wasn't.

But back then, no one would've known.

Because high performers don't break.

They just burn quieter. And I was burning.

The weird part is, I didn't think I was traumatized. I thought I was doing what men are supposed to do. Keep going. Push through. Don't make it about you. That kind of thing.

But the guilt crawled in slowly.

I kept asking myself: *Why him and not me? He was better than me. He had more to give. Why the hell am I still here?*

I didn't have words for it back then. I still don't have all of them. But I know what it did. It made me smaller inside. Quieter. It turned off parts of me I used to like.

And I kept pretending everything was fine. Smiling at the right times. Making jokes. Getting promotions. Being the guy who always had the tools, always had the answers.

No one teaches you how to grieve. Especially not men like me, from families like mine.

So, I buried the fear, the anger, the sadness. I buried it all under routines and responsibilities. Until the weight of it all became too much to carry.

But that was before. Before I was diagnosed. Before I even knew what PTSD really was.

It started here. In the silence. In the stuff I never said.

But there was a moment. A specific day that carved itself into me. The moment I now see as the point where everything started to unravel quietly.

It was July 2007. My birthday.

The ship was carving lazy search patterns through the Florida Straits, water flat as glass, sun already heavy overhead. I had the early morning watch, half-awake but wired in that way you are when you're running on routine and fumes.

It didn't take long before we spotted something. A vessel on the horizon. Barely twenty-three feet, maybe, and overloaded, with at least forty people onboard. Cuban migrants trying to make it to the US to seek asylum. Families. Men. Women. Kids.

The captain gave the order to launch the small boat. I was the coxswain.

We sped toward the boat, closing fast, radios crackling with urgency. It was brutally hot, thick air, no shade, sun beating down on bare metal and skin. As we approached, the yelling started. Spanish, fast and panicked, overlapping voices coming from their boat and ours. I didn't understand most of it.

Neither did my crew. Just fragments, words that felt urgent, scared, defiant.

One man stood up, a child clutched in front of him. He poured what looked like gasoline from a bottle, soaking them both, and held a lighter high in the air.

His fingers shook. The kid, who couldn't have been more than four, clung to his leg, face pressed into denim. Gasoline slicked both their skin. It smelled like the garage back home. Like the cans I'd stacked beside the lawnmower. Like something normal turned into a weapon.

This was my first op back after Jay. One person buried, two more about to burn.

A voice crackled on the radio. "Back off, Pat. He's gonna do it."

I didn't move. Engine idling. Water slapping the hull. Sun drilling into my neck.

The kid peeked out. Dark eyes. Wide. Not scared yet, just curious.

I raised my hand, palm out. "No mas!"

Time didn't slow. It shattered.

Jay's laugh on the golf course.

The thud of the golf ball hitting his skull.

"Nobody ever got hurt sitting on the couch."

My throat locked. Not fear. Fury. At him. At me. At the whole fucked-up math that said this kid's life was worth less than a line on a map.

"Turn around!" someone shouted from the bow. "Goddamn it, turn!"

I wrenched the throttle. Spray hit my face. Salt and shame.

When I looked back, there was no flame. The man slumped. The kid stared at me over his shoulder.

I'd see those eyes for years. In the shower. At the dinner table. In the silence between Lizzie's breaths.

We'd attempt to stop them no less than three more times. Every time we got close, the same thing happened: the bottle, the lighter, the kid.

Over and over. The man wanted us to know he was willing to do it. And we believed him.

Finally, another cutter got in range with a prop entanglement device and deployed it cleanly. Their engine locked up, and the boat stopped.

We came alongside, and the migrants couldn't get off their boat fast enough, scrambling to reach us, crawling over one another to climb aboard. We pulled every last person out of that boat. And when it was empty, we sank it.

The next morning, ICE agents showed up and quietly removed three human smugglers from the group.

And that was that.

Paperwork. Debriefs. A few jokes. Maybe a birthday wish or two.

But inside, I was wrecked. The image of that kid's eyes was seared onto the back of my eyelids. I kept seeing Jay's face, as well. One life lost to the water, another almost sacrificed to it. The same helplessness, the same silent scream caught in my chest.

That night, the crew surprised me. With a few tired smiles and a nod of recognition, they brought out a Boston cream pie. They'd radioed ahead and had the galley save it.

I stared at it. The perfect swirls of chocolate frosting. The dumb, beautiful normalcy of it. As if nothing had happened. As if today were just another day.

I took a bite. In a world that kept spinning on its axis while I was still trying to find my footing on the deck, it tasted like ash and salt.

Chapter Three
FAR FROM PERFECT

On the surface, everything looked fine. Normal. Solid even. I left the Coast Guard with an honorable discharge, married my sweetheart a year later, and we quickly settled into our life together. I showed up. I worked. I provided. I made sure the kids were fed, that bills were paid, that I made it to hockey games. But inside? I was cooked. Burned out and still burning.

For a while I told myself it was age. *You're getting older, man. That's all it is.* I blamed the fatigue, the headaches, and the brain fog on time catching up with me. Then I thought maybe it was ADHD, thought I was bipolar or depressed, thought I was something, anything. Got tested, even tried the meds.

They didn't work. Just made the noise louder. The problem wasn't focus. It was the weight. The kind you can't name but still carry.

I was gone and didn't even know it. Dissociating. Living life ten feet behind my own eyes. I'd be mid-conversation and forget where I was. I'd drive home and have zero memory of the route. I'd walk into a room and forget why. Normal stuff, I guess, until it wasn't.

Lizzie saw it. She always sees it. I don't know how, but she just knows when I'm off. She'd step in before I blew. Quietly take over. Guide the kids away from me like it was part of the nightly routine. I'd stomp around like I had a right to be angry. Like the world owed me peace, and I hadn't earned it yet.

One night, Flynn spilled juice on the floor. A nothing moment. But I snapped. Not violent. Just loud. Sharp. Enough to change the room. Mairin bolted to the toy room. Declan cleaned it up without a word. Lizzie just stood there and took it in. No yelling. No lecture. Just a look. And in that look was everything I hated about myself.

Later that night, we crawled into bed. She didn't say much. Just whispered, "You don't have to carry all of it." I didn't respond. What was I gonna say? I don't even know what "it" is?

But it got worse.

Headaches. Tight chest. Always on edge. I'd wake up sweating from dreams I couldn't remember, and I'd feel like I hadn't slept at all.

It was a Saturday, but there's no such thing as rest days in my house. Not really. By 8:53 a.m., the house was already alive with full-blown mayhem. Mairin was blasting Taylor Swift in the living room. Declan was rifling through the mudroom yelling about a missing elbow pad. Flynn was half-naked, running laps with a plastic sword, occasionally whacking the dog and screaming "hi-*ya!*" at the top of his lungs. Lizzie was at the stove, flipping pancakes with one hand and holding her coffee like it was a lifeline with the other.

And me?

I was standing in the kitchen, holding an empty mug, trying to remember if I'd already made the coffee or just thought about it.

My head was pounding. My back hurt. I hadn't even taken a sip of water yet. Not enough caffeine or weed in the world to dull the edges of that morning. The noise wasn't just noise. It was pressure. Like the house itself was closing in. Every sound felt personal. Every bump, scream, spill, screech like it was being aimed right at the base of my skull.

I wasn't angry, exactly.

I was . . . overloaded, overstimulated.

My jaw was clenched, shoulders tight, fists balled without even realizing it.

Lizzie looked over, calm somehow.

"You good?" she asked, like she already knew the answer.

I nodded. Lied. "Yeah. Just tired."

I hadn't stopped drinking at first, I just paired it with weed. I'd get cross-faded more than I'd like to admit. There were nights I couldn't remember how I got to bed, but I told myself I had it under control. I told Lizzie the same thing. I think we both knew better.

That Christmas, I stumbled into the side of the house. Cracked my face against the doorframe and gave myself a black eye. Woke up the next morning trying to pretend it didn't happen. The kids saw. Lizzie didn't say much. She didn't have to.

Later that week, she told me flat out: I had to pick one. I couldn't keep doing both. I couldn't keep being this version of myself.

So I chose the weed. Told myself it was the lesser evil. That it helped with the nerves, the sleep, the noise. And for a little while, it did.

I was sober for maybe a year. No booze, anyway. But I wasn't better. Just dulled.

Then came Jamaica. A family trip. It should've been nothing but sun and ocean and watching the kids play in the sand. But I let my guard down. Had a drink. Then another. Then whatever invisible line I thought I'd built around myself washed away with the tide.

I lost my temper. Snapped at Lizzie over something small. Something I can't even remember now. What I do remember is the look on her face. And how close I came to losing everything.

That was the second decision. The real one. I gave up drinking for good after that. I've been sober ever since.

But the damage was done. I didn't feel like a husband anymore. Not really. Not the kind I wanted to be. I was a presence in the house, but I wasn't present. The kids brought home drawings and trophies and stories. I smiled, nodded, and disappeared into myself.

The anger didn't go away. It just got quieter. More poisonous. I'd snap over spilled juice or slammed doors. I could see the way they braced for it. Like waiting for lightning to strike. I hated that version of me. But I didn't know how to stop being him.

At the rink, I'd stand with the other dads. Cheer like I was supposed to. But I'd blink and the game would be over. No memory of it. Just this hollow ache, like I'd missed something important but couldn't rewind the tape.

After one of Declan's games, Lizzie said, "He was looking for you in the stands. Wanted to make sure you saw the goal."

I said I did but I hadn't.

At one game, I had been on edge before I even got to the rink. Then I saw who would officiate. I swear this one ref had it out for me. Or maybe it was mutual by that point. I won't pretend I'm the bigger man here. Every time he was assigned to one of our games, my stomach tightened. He missed the most obvious calls—blatant hooks, slashes, and holds—and then would whistle kids for borderline offsides like it was the Stanley Cup Final. It was like he wanted to be part of the game, not call it. This game, I'd had enough. He missed three straight calls, all against us. Kids were getting frustrated. I was fuming. Finally, I said to him, loud enough for the stands to hear...

"I can't believe you get paid to be this bad at your job."

He tossed me without hesitation. Finger pointing, red in the face, his voice cracking like puberty had returned just to fuel the drama. Honestly? Worth it. It was a good line. Still makes me laugh. But even then, beneath the sarcasm, I knew it wasn't about the ref.

Not really.

Looking back, I was constantly bringing that weight to the rink. Thought I left it at home, but it followed me everywhere. I yelled at practices. Pushed the kids harder than I needed to. Demanded focus, demanded perfection, but I was nowhere close to perfect myself. I'd blow up over missed passes, bad positioning, lazy backchecks. It was never really about hockey. It was about me. My failure to hold things together. My own cracks showing up in their ice time.

I'd slam the bench door when we got scored on. Loud. Angry. Not at the kids, but they felt it anyway. I know they did. I still see the way they looked down after mistakes, how some of them stopped celebrating goals like they used to. That joy . . . I dulled it.

There were games where I couldn't even look them in the eye afterward. Not because of the loss but because I knew I'd made it heavier. Because I'd coached like a man who was trying to win something deeper than a trophy. I was trying to win back control of a life that was slipping. And I used the game to do it. That was never fair to them.

The scary part is I thought I was hiding it. Thought I was doing a decent job. Suit up. Show up. Smile for the camera. But everyone felt it. Especially Lizzie. She'd been carrying my dead weight for years, and I didn't even realize it.

One night, we were on the couch. Kids were asleep. Glass of wine in her hand, TV on but muted. She looked over and said, "I miss you."

I didn't even know how to respond. I was sitting right next to her, but she was right, I wasn't really there.

"I know," I said.

She nodded. "I know you do."

That's the kind of love people don't write enough about. The love that doesn't flinch when it hurts.

My temper was short. My fuse was fried. Things that never used to bother me would set me off. I'd slam doors, snap at Lizzie. That dead-eyed stare into nothing. And every time I lost it, I promised I'd do better.

Sometimes I did. Most times I didn't.

The kids knew the signs. It wasn't when I'd yell but when the room went still. They'd scatter when I got quiet. They didn't tiptoe out of fear. They moved like they were giving me space. Like I was a pressure cooker about to rupture.

And Lizzie, God, she never made it about her. But she carried everything. The schedules. The meals. The moods. Mine especially.

That woman's a lighthouse. And I kept crashing into the rocks anyway.

I still thought I could carry it all. Thought I could bury grief under routine. Thought showing up meant something. Thought pretending was protecting them.

I didn't know it yet, but this was just the opening act.

The storm was still gathering.

And it was coming straight for me.

Chapter Four
The Four Corners of Me

RANNON—the Foundation

He came first. I was twenty. Barely holding my own shit together and still living in a shared apartment in Rockland with a couple other guys; one of them was Jonas, who became my best friend. Coast Guard pay, a busted futon, and duct tape on half the stuff I owned.

His mom and I weren't together. We tried, but it wasn't built to last. He came fast, born in Portland with a bilateral cleft lip and pallet. The Rockland hospital couldn't handle the delivery, so we rushed south. I remember the drive like it was yesterday. Everything felt like it was spinning.

And then he was here. My son. Small. Fragile. Face stitched with this line of imperfection that somehow made him more perfect than anything I'd ever seen. I remember holding him, not knowing what the hell I was supposed to do next. But something inside me clicked.

I wasn't ready to be a dad, but I was one. And that was that.

Those first few years were a grind. Surgeries. Appointments. Specialty bottles that looked like lab equipment. I'd rock him in that shitty apartment while my roommates played video games in the next room. It was chaos. But it was ours.

He was on base constantly. Everyone knew Rannon. Bundled up in the Maine cold, wide eyes, quiet. The kid who didn't cry much. Just watched. Took it all in.

Later, when I got transferred to Woods Hole, his mom moved back to Nebraska. But Rannon still came out to see me. First on weekends then for whole summers. We built something out of those trips, just the two of us. No script. No perfect plan. Just effort. I never forced anything. I just made sure he knew I was always there.

And the crazy thing is, he kept coming back. Even when he got older, even when he had a life out there, he still wanted to be with me. That tells you everything about him.

He doesn't need much. Doesn't make noise. But that silence? I know it too well. I wore it for years. It's not peace. It's armor.

He's steady. Smart. Not loud, but present. He sees more than he says. I catch it in the way he looks at his siblings. In the way he asks about my day. In the way he never bailed, even when he had every reason to.

He never needed me to be perfect. He just needed me to show up. And somehow, even when I was falling apart, I did. Not always well. Not always clean. But I was there. And so was he.

He was the first one to make me believe I could be a father. Not just a provider. Not just a guy who signs paperwork and sends birthday gifts. A real father. That's why he's the foundation. Because everything I built after him, every kid, every move, every second chance, I built on the ground he helped me find.

DECLAN—the Firekeeper

Declan's got my engine. Always has. Runs hot, never lets up, never sits still. Even when he was little, he didn't walk, he charged. Not angry. Just determined. Like he had something to prove, even if nobody was asking.

He's not the biggest kid. Never was. Got cut from teams that didn't think he had enough. I watched him take those hits and come back harder every time. He doesn't say much about it, but I know the feeling. I gave him that feeling. That need to show you belong.

I coached him for ten straight years. Every season. Every practice. Every stupid, cold rink at 5:30 in the morning. I tied his skates; I yelled from the bench; I watched him grow into himself shift by shift. This coming season will be the first time I'm not behind the bench with him. Still not sure how I feel about that.

That Peewee year he was twelve, that was a war. Team got bounced from State in a heartbreaker, one of those games where the air leaves the room, and nobody moves for a full minute after the buzzer. Crushed them. But a few weeks later, they rallied and won Regionals. No one saw that coming.

Declan started to rise during that stretch. Not just on the scoresheet, but in the room. He stopped being just a player. Started becoming a presence. A kid the others looked to. That's when I knew: He had something.

He's on track now to play high school hockey his freshman season. That blows my mind. I never even touched JV or varsity. I was barely hanging on to the practice squad. He's already miles ahead of where I ever was, and he's only just getting started.

But that same season, while he was catching fire, I was burning out.

That was the year we lost my dad. Dementia finally took him. The writing had been on the wall, but I didn't, or wouldn't, see it. So, when it happened, it felt fast. Like I blinked and he was gone.

I was in the room when he passed. I didn't want to be. I told myself I didn't need to be. But I was. I saw him take his last breath. I heard my mother cry. I heard my sister call out "Dad" with a voice I'll never forget. I wanted so badly to run, to walk out and pretend I didn't hear any of it.

But I didn't move.

Declan was at hockey that night. My wife took him. I stayed back with my father as he left this world.

And that's what makes this all so damn complicated.

On the outside, I was the proud dad, coaching his son to Regionals, getting him ready for the next level. On the inside, I was losing mine, watching the man who raised me slip away piece by piece . . . and then all at once.

I don't know if Declan knows how much of me broke that year. I hope not. I don't want to hang that weight on him.

But every time he steps on the ice, I see it. The fight. The fire. The way he keeps going, even when it hurts.

That's how I know he's mine.

MAIRIN—the Soul Guide

She's the only girl. The only one who can look me dead in the eye, tilt her head just a little, and undo every defense I've spent a lifetime building.

There's something ancient about her. Like she came here already knowing too much. She reads energy. She senses tone shifts. If I walk in the room pretending I'm okay, she knows before I say a word.

And she's only eight.

She still calls me "Dada." I hope she never stops. That little voice cracks me in half. Doesn't matter what mood I'm in—rage, grief, shut down, spinning—she cuts right through it.

She's got this way of existing that's soft but not fragile. Curious, but clear. She asks the kind of questions that stop me cold. Not to be a smartass. Just because she wants to understand the world, and she wants me to help her do it.

But some days . . . some days I can't help. Some days I'm too far gone in my own storm. And those are the days that break me.

Because she doesn't get mad. She gets quiet.

There was one night I snapped. Nothing huge, just one of those dumb moments that come from being overstimulated, tired, stretched too thin. I slammed a door. Just loud enough to rattle the walls. And she disappeared. I found her later in the toy room, tucked into the corner, holding her stuffed animal like a shield.

She didn't cry. She didn't even look scared.

She looked disappointed.

Like part of her thought I was better than that. And I had to sit with that. Still do.

I've spent my whole life trying to be strong, trying to protect people. But here's my daughter, eight years old, teaching me that real strength is knowing when to soften. When to feel instead of fight.

And God help me, she melts me. Every single day.

She could look me in the eye, confess to murder, and I'd be out back digging the hole before she finished the sentence. That's not a joke. That's just the gravitational pull she has on me.

She doesn't need saving. She never has. What she needs is me—present, regulated, real. Not the version that's armored up or hiding in busyness. The me that listens. The me that sees her.

And when I can get out of my own way, that version shows up.

She pulls it out of me. Gently. Patiently.

That's why she's the soul guide. When I forget who I am, she reminds me. Not with words. With presence.

And if I ever do anything right in this life, it'll be making sure the world doesn't crush that light in her.

Because I know what it means to lose yourself trying to survive, and I'll be damned if that's her story.

FLYNN—the Disruptor, the Healer

Flynn wasn't planned. Not by the calendar. Not by the budget. Not by anything resembling logic. But the second the test turned positive, something in me knew this one's coming for a reason.

He showed up like a wrecking ball in the best way. Loud, wild, a tiny human tornado that doesn't walk, just collides. And somehow, that chaos brought a calm with it. Doesn't make sense, I know. But that's Flynn. Nothing about him fits the mold, and none of it needs to.

He was born at a time when I didn't think I had much left to give. I was worn out. Physically, mentally, emotionally. I had nothing in the tank, and then this little beast came screaming into the world as if to say, "Get up, Dad."

And I did.

Because there was no other option.

At three years old, he's already everything I'm still trying to be. Present. Joyful. Unfiltered. He's a full-body laugh and a deep-sigh nap. He makes a mess and doesn't apologize for it. He demands to be held when he needs comfort and doesn't pretend otherwise.

I wish I was that honest with myself.

The bond between Flynn and my mom caught me off guard. She watches him a couple days a week now, and I swear he's keeping her alive. She lives for it, for him. There's something about the way he looks at her, like he already knows she's been through the fire and came out still standing. It's not just a nana thing. It's deeper. Soul stuff.

And when my dad was dying, Flynn was the only one who could get a smile out of him. Last few months, barely responsive ... and then Flynn would waddle in, babbling nonsense, and there it was. A flicker. A lift. A reason.

One soul coming in while another was heading out.

I don't think that was an accident.

Flynn is the reminder that life doesn't stop. That something always follows the silence. That maybe the end of one chapter can still open into joy if you're willing to hold on a little longer.

He's only three. But I swear, he's already cracked me wide open in a way nothing else has.

He didn't just arrive to be loved.

He arrived to teach me how to love again.

Chapter Five

CRACKS IN THE ICE

I started coaching Declan when he was just a Mite. He might've barely known how to skate, but he had a fire from the beginning. We'd hit the ice early, sometimes before the sun was even up, and I swear he never once complained. He just loved it. We ran three-on-three games, half-ice chaos, puck touches everywhere. Kids falling over each other, giggling, losing sticks, scoring on the wrong net. It wasn't about systems or structure back then; it was just pure joy. Unfiltered hockey joy.

Those early years I wasn't "Coach Lyons," I was just Dad. Just some guy with beat-up skates and a bag full of cones, trying to make sure every kid left the rink smiling. We kept it light. I'd crack jokes during drills, challenge them to races, let them play knee hockey in the locker room until someone inevitably banged their head on a bench. We had something good back then. Something real. Hockey was the place where we laughed the most. Where we bonded without trying. I wish I could have held on to what we had longer. I wish I hadn't let the pressure, the expectations, the storm in my head leak into the rink. Because back then, the rink was the safest place I knew.

When Declan hit Squirts, we made the decision he'd play both town and club. Not because we were chasing anything, but because he wanted to play on a team I didn't coach. I think he needed space to find himself as a player, not just as "Coach's kid." And honestly? I needed it too. I didn't know that then, but looking back, I can see it. That was the beginning of something shifting. The start of the weight creeping in.

We had made it to the state finals that first year in Pee-wees. That alone should've been enough. For the kids, for the parents, for me. But we didn't win. We fought hard, gave everything we had, but the scoreboard didn't swing our way. I'll never forget the faces in the room afterward. Red eyes, gear strewn on the floor, silence so thick it pressed in from every corner. I stood in the middle of it all, trying to say the right thing, trying to keep it together.

The worst part? I think I took it harder than any of them.

I wanted to be strong, the way coaches are supposed to be. But inside I was breaking down. And the universe, in its twisted sense of humor, gave us more hockey to play. Regionals were the following week.

The ride home was long. Quiet. Crushing. I didn't even play music. Just me and the road and a head full of thoughts I couldn't outrun. Friends called, texted. *How excited are you to go back to the rink after that loss?* someone joked. I laughed. Or at least, I typed *lol*. But the truth? I wasn't excited. I was drained. Numb.

The Monday after States was brutal. I fielded some angry phone calls, but they were mostly just from raw disappointment that we'd lost. The tone wasn't one of support or perspective. It was finger-pointing. There had been an expectation we'd take it all. And when we didn't, someone had to carry that blame. That someone was me.

Practice that week felt like walking barefoot across broken glass. The air was heavy, the locker room silent. I screamed at Declan one night, really screamed at him, for being late to get on the ice. I made the whole team skate suicides because of it. I stood there, whistle in my hand, watching them gasp for air, and a voice in my head, quiet but clear, broke through the rage:

Who are you to punish these kids?

They are kids. They just laid everything they had on the ice for you. For each other. They played their hearts out and they lost, and now you're making them pay for your own failure. For your own shame that you can't fucking outskate.

Look at them. You're breaking it. That thing in them that loves this game. That joy. You're the one with the whistle, and you're breaking it.

I wanted to scream at myself to stop. To blow the whistle and call them in and tell them I was sorry, that I was wrong, that it was me, not them. But I didn't. I just stood there, my jaw locked, my heart hammering with a shame so deep it felt like drowning. I had become the very thing I hated—a bully with a clipboard, using their effort as a whetstone to sharpen my own self-loathing.

Declan took it. So did the rest of the kids. And I hated myself for it. The truth is, I still hate myself for it.

I've replayed that moment a thousand times. I've tried to bury it under years of other games, other practices, other apologies. But it sits in me, a cold, hard stone of shame. I wasn't just a coach having a bad day. I was a man who was supposed to protect that joy, and instead, I took a hammer to it. I looked at a group of kids who had given me everything they had, kids who weren't even mine to break, and I used their effort to punish myself. I became the exact thing I promised I'd never be.

I don't know if I can ever forgive myself for that. Some things are too big for forgiveness. Some mistakes don't fade; they just become a part of who you are. A reminder, etched in bone, of the cost of falling apart and the people who pay the price when you do. Not my best moment. Not even close.

Then came Regionals. A second chance, but I was still carrying the weight. We opened Friday night against the Connecticut state champs and lost. Some part of me, deep down, almost wanted that to happen. Like, *You wanted fair? You wanted equal ice time? Here you go.* I didn't tank the game, but I didn't fight for it either. I was still so angry, at myself, at the parents, at everything.

Saturday was different. We went up against the Massachusetts state champions in the semifinals. They jumped out to a 5-0 lead by the second period. It looked like our ride was over. But the boys, God, those boys, they didn't quit. They stormed back with six unanswered goals. I watched it unfold like a man waking up from a long sleep. We were alive. And the locker room afterward? That was the closest I'd felt to joy in a long time.

That comeback lined us up against Darien, Connecticut in the final. Back and forth game. A battle. One of the best I'd ever seen them play. They earned every shift, every shot, every backcheck. They played their hearts out. And I was so damn proud. Still am.

Half the town showed up for that final. I'm not exaggerating. There was a full-on student section led by the high school varsity hockey team, banging the glass, waving signs, chanting every name like it was the Bruins' Cup run. It felt electric. A sea of people who believed. That rink hadn't seen noise like that in years, maybe ever. The kids fed off it. The energy was unreal. For the first time all season, I saw joy without baggage. Competition without fear. And for one fleeting moment, I let myself feel proud, an undiluted, unfiltered pride in them and in myself, too.

After the final horn, I watched them dogpile on the ice, helmets flying. The pure joy in that moment, it almost made me believe again.

Almost...

We made history that weekend. It was everything you hope a season can become. But for me, the high didn't hold.

That Regionals win lifted me, sure, but only for a short time.

That whole season was a roller coaster. It was also the year my dad passed. I probably should've seen it coming, but I didn't. I refused to. When it happened, it felt sudden, even though the signs had been there. I didn't talk about it. Just shoved it down and kept moving. That grief was in the air all season long, and I never once named it.

I kept thinking about Declan. About the other kids. About how they deserved someone better in that moment . . .

Looking back now, it was all there, the signs, the symptoms, the fallout. I thought coaching would be the thing that saved me. But it was also the mirror that showed me just how far I'd drifted.

The victory didn't reset anything. If anything, it exposed how far gone I really was.

I started to wonder why I felt this way. Why even winning didn't feel like a win. Why the highs weren't lifting me and the lows were digging trenches. Why I'd built all of this up as if coaching these kids would somehow save me, and why I still felt so fucking lost.

It wasn't just about hockey. It hadn't been for a while.

That's when it hit me. I needed help. Not a break. Not a vacation. Real help.

Back then, I wasn't in therapy yet, at least not the kind that gets to the root. I had started seeing a psychiatrist, referred by my PCP. But it felt clinical, almost transactional. We talked about anxiety. We talked about depression. We talked about everything. But PTSD wasn't on the table, not because he missed it but because I didn't present it. The symptoms hadn't lined up in a way that pointed to trauma. I wasn't talking about hypervigilance or nightmares or emotional numbness. I was talking about focus issues. Restlessness. Trouble finishing tasks. I thought I was burned out or maybe just wired wrong. He treated what I brought into the room. That's not on him. That's how pain works; it wears different masks until, one day, it doesn't.

I'd made it through years thinking I was just tired or moody. But this wasn't just stress. This was something that had rooted deep in my bones, something that bled into my coaching, my marriage, my fatherhood.

And still, I kept showing up. That was the most brutal part. Not the pain, not the exhaustion, just the pretending.

Pretending I had this under control. Pretending the win had fixed something. Pretending I wasn't one hard question away from losing it all.

HOLD FAST

There's a loneliness in that kind of pretending. You get good at masks. You forget how to take them off.

Chapter Six
BLEEDING IN

I wasn't suicidal.

Not in the way people think. I wasn't standing on the bridge or counting pills or writing goodbye letters.

But I also wasn't okay. Every night was a prayer. I would lie in bed, eyes clenched shut, and wish for it. Not to kill myself but to simply cease. I would pray to whatever might be listening, God, the universe, the empty dark, to just take me while I slept. To make it painless. To make it final. And under my breath, a hum, a desperate, silent mantra against the pillow:

I wanna die I wanna die I wanna die.

A lullaby for the damned on a loop until exhaustion finally pulled me under. And every morning when the sun hit the window and I realized I was still here; the first feeling wasn't relief. It was a deep, hollow disappointment. Another day to get through.

Every day I felt heavier. Numb. Like I was slowly disappearing under the weight of my own life.

I had already fallen apart in more ways than I was willing to admit—lost it at work, scared my kids, scared myself. And now I couldn't even get a callback.

I tried. Called around. Asked for help. Left voicemails. Every provider had a waitlist. Every psych referral led to an automated message or a receptionist telling me to try back in six months.

Unless I was in crisis.

Then I could be seen immediately. That was the system.

So, I told them what I had to. I said the words that would open the door. I said, "I'm not safe." And maybe that was true in a way I hadn't let myself admit yet.

That was how I got into outpatient.

Cape Cod Hospital. Fluorescent lights. Coffee that tasted like hot tin. Folding chairs around a table in a beige room. The clock on the wall ticked too loud. I had a badge with my name on it and a group session schedule that felt more like detention than healing.

I walked in with my guard all the way up. Sat in the corner, arms folded. Watched the room like I was still standing quarterdeck watch. Everyone else looked like they belonged there. People detoxing. People just released from inpatient. People who had been dragged back from the edge and weren't sure how to live now that they were still here.

And me? I felt like a fake. Like I was wasting a seat. Like I was taking resources away from someone worse off. But I stayed. I kept showing up. I didn't talk much. I listened.

Some people were loud. Angry. Twitchy. Some were so soft-spoken I could barely hear them. A few cracked jokes that were only funny if you'd ever been on the edge of the abyss and looked down. They talked about panic, relapse, flashbacks, isolation. About the things they lost and the versions of themselves they missed.

What I heard in that room opened something inside of me. Not all at once. Not a breakthrough. But a slow shift. A realization from somewhere down deep: *You are not the only one bleeding in silence.*

Eventually, I met with a psychiatric NP. She was older. Wore those wire-framed glasses that made her look both too smart and too tired. She asked good questions. Listened in a way that felt uncomfortable at first, like I didn't know how to be seen for who I was without flinching.

We talked meds. Risks. Side effects. Options. I walked out with a prescription and a skeptical shrug. I wasn't sure I believed in the meds; they hadn't worked before, but I took them. Didn't miss a day.

I started to feel . . . something. Not better. But a little more like a person. A little less like a landmine waiting to go off. Like the volume knob on the chaos in my head had been turned down just enough for me to breathe.

Outpatient didn't fix me. But it bought me time. It gave me structure. It forced me to sit still long enough to realize I was still alive. I wasn't okay, but I wasn't beyond repair.

There was a Tuesday morning group that always started with silence. Nobody wanted to speak first. The air would just hang there, stale. One guy, Rick, would usually be the one to finally break the silence, say something dark or sarcastic to get a laugh. He reminded me of guys I knew in the service. Tough exterior, shattered inside. We never exchanged numbers. Never hung out. But I still think about him. I think about all of them. Because for a few hours a week, we were in the same boat. Bailing water with our hands, trying not to sink.

Outpatient forced me to slow down long enough to see the wreckage. Not just the wreckage I caused but the wreckage I'd become. My nervous system was fried, my patience gone. My brain felt like a buzzing power line with frayed edges. I couldn't remember the last time I laughed without forcing it.

Still, I almost quit. Twice. Once after a group session where someone shared something about losing a sibling that hit too close to home. I wanted to bolt. Wanted to scream that I didn't belong there. But instead, I clenched my jaw, stared at the wall, and counted to sixty over and over again until the urge passed.

I'm glad I stayed.

I won't pretend that every session was a revelation or helped me. A lot of it felt like recycled advice, with clinical handouts and jargon that bounced off my skull. But underneath all that, something was happening. Some quiet, invisible repair. A recalibration.

I stopped checking out as often. I started noticing things. The smell of coffee in the morning. The way Mairin curled up on the couch with her stuffed animals. The way Lizzie still looked at me, even when I didn't deserve it.

That felt new. And it mattered.

But I think it was that first group session that got to me.

We were in a circle, the kind that makes you feel like a middle schooler at a trust-building seminar. The facilitator, a woman named Sam, a social worker by trade, voice soft, started with, "Anyone want to share how they're feeling walking in today?"

Silence.

A woman next to me picked at the label on her water bottle until it shredded. A guy across from me, Mark, I'd learn later, just stared at the wall. Finally, someone spoke. A kid, maybe twenty-one, tattoos up his neck and eyes that looked a decade older. "I feel like shit, man. Like I don't even know who I am anymore."

I nodded, instinctively, then froze, like I'd given something away.

When it came around to me, I said something generic. "Just . . . trying to figure some stuff out." That was my go-to. Vague. Neutral. Not enough to invite follow-ups.

Sam didn't push. Just nodded and moved on. But something in me noticed the quiet acceptance of it. No one asked me to justify my pain. No one questioned if I deserved to be there. And for the first time in months, I didn't feel like I had to defend my right to be hurting.

They handed out journals that day. Little black composition books with our names written in Sharpie on the front. "Try to write in it at least once a day," Sam said. "Doesn't have to be deep. Just honest."

I didn't write that night. I stared at the page. I thought about writing to Jay. I thought about writing to Lizzie. But it all felt forced. Instead, I drew lines. Thick, overlapping black lines. Angry ones. That was enough.

Week two, things started to surface. One woman talked about her son, how he wouldn't speak to her anymore. Another guy shared how he couldn't go grocery shopping without having a panic attack in the dairy aisle. Something about the lights, the cold, the pressure of decision-making. I got that. The places where anxiety hides, those aren't the moments people don't warn you about.

One afternoon, I left group and drove to the harbor. I parked by the docks and just sat there in my truck, engine off, staring at the water. Everything was moving—boats rocking, gulls circling, flags flapping—but I was still. Paralyzed. I started breathing fast. Too fast. Vision narrowing. Chest getting tight. I tried to ground myself. I counted boats, traced the dashboard with my thumb, but it didn't help. I gripped the steering wheel like it was a lifeline.

I don't know how long I sat there like that. But when I finally came back to myself, my face was wet. Silent tears. I wasn't even aware they had started.

That night, I wrote in the journal.

I am not okay. I don't know when that started being true, but I know it now.

That felt like progress.

We had a worksheet one day with examples of cognitive distortions. Black-and-white thinking. Catastrophizing. Emotional reasoning. Each one read like a personal description.

If I'm not perfect, I'm a failure.
If something bad can happen, it will.
If I feel it, it must be true.

I looked up from the page and half laughed. "Did they write this just for me?"

Sam smiled. "No, but it's scary how close it hits, huh?"

She gave me an extra printout. I taped it to the fridge at home, just to see if Lizzie would notice. She did. She didn't say anything. Just circled three of them and left it there.

After three weeks in, I noticed my posture had changed. I wasn't folding my arms as much. Wasn't scanning the room like I was about to be attacked. I was listening. Sometimes even nodding. I still wasn't sharing much, but I was present.

One day in group, a woman broke down in the middle of the room. Sobbing. Couldn't speak. I felt something in me rise, instinct maybe. I slid her a tissue box across the floor like we were back in kindergarten. She looked up and whispered, "Thanks," like it meant the world. That wrecked me. Because I knew how much courage it took to just . . . be seen.

Outside of group, things were still hard. One night I got home, and Mairin showed me a picture she'd drawn. It was our family, again. But this time, I was there, in the corner, holding her hand.

She looked up at me and said, "That's us on the deck. You're smiling."

I choked on that smile. I held it together, kissed her head, thanked her. Later, I stared at that drawing for twenty minutes. I hadn't smiled in months. Not really. But maybe she was showing me something I couldn't yet see in myself.

The meds started to level out my energy. I wasn't wired. I wasn't sedated. Just . . . less jagged. The edges softened. I could handle the grocery store without sweating through my shirt. I could sit through a meeting without my leg bouncing like a jackhammer. The fog hadn't lifted, but I could see my hand in front of my face again.

At one point in group, we were asked to name something we missed about ourselves.

I said, "The version of me that used to sing in the car."

It came out before I even thought about it. And it landed hard because I couldn't remember the last time I'd done that, windows down, music up, just letting it fly.

That became a small goal. Not a stretch, not therapy homework, just a personal flag. One night, driving home from outpatient, I put on an old song Jay used to love and I sang. Quiet at first. Then louder. It cracked and wavered and choked, but it came out. I was still in there somewhere.

I think that's what healing really is. Not becoming someone new. Just remembering who you were before the weight.

It would take almost two more years before someone gave me the word for what I was dealing with. But outpatient was the moment I stopped pretending I was fine. It was the first time I realized that naming the storm doesn't calm it, but it might keep you from drowning in it.

Outpatient gave me that first glimpse. Not the full picture. But enough to hold onto.

Enough to bleed in the storm and stay standing.

Chapter Seven
THE DISAPPEARING ACT

I used to be the guy who filled rooms. Loud laugh. Strong opinions. Always had a story, usually too long and way too detailed. I was the coach. The funny one. The guy people leaned on. The guy people called. And then, somehow, I became the guy nobody noticed had gone missing.

You don't realize how fast it happens. One excuse turns into two. Two into a pattern. The pattern becomes who you are.

I remember one night when Lizzie came home from a neighborhood thing. I don't even remember what it was, someone's birthday party maybe. She walked in, took off her shoes, and just looked at me.

"You used to love these things," she said. Not accusing. Just tired. "They ask about you. But it's like you're already gone."

She didn't say it to hurt me. But it did. Because she was right. I wasn't there anymore. Not in the way that mattered. And the worst part? I didn't know how to come back. I'd been gone too long.

I avoided even the people I missed. Guys I would've killed to grab a beer with I ghosted. Not because I didn't care but because I cared too much. Because the idea of pretending I was okay for a whole night felt impossible.

I didn't want to lie anymore. Didn't want to smile when I didn't mean it. Didn't want to be "on." So, I stayed "off." All the time.

There were moments when I'd think, *Okay, today I'll go. I'll show up. I'll get dressed. I'll rally.* But then the time would come, and I'd feel that familiar weight in my chest. That pressure in my head. Like someone pressing down on my sternum with a cold, heavy hand.

And I'd cave. Again.

There were also things I wanted to say. Honest things, like "I'm sorry I keep bailing. I'm not okay," or "I want to see you, but I'm drowning." But those things never made it past my lips.

Instead, I'd text *Sorry, can't make it tonight* or, worse, not respond at all.

That's the thing about PTSD. It's not just the panic or the rage or the flashbacks. Sometimes it's the numbness. The withdrawal. The disappearing act. People think if you're not in crisis, you must be okay.

But what if the crisis is that you don't feel anything at all?

There was a point where I realized even my own kids had started adapting to my absence. They stopped asking me to go places. If there was a family walk, they'd just leave without me. If they had a school event, Lizzie would be the one in the photos. I'd be at home, telling myself I needed to rest, that I wasn't up for it.

And every time I missed one of those moments, a part of me cracked a little deeper.

One night, Mairin came into the living room with a drawing she'd made. It showed her, her brothers, and Lizzie standing outside in the sun. I wasn't in it. I asked her why.

She shrugged. "You were sleeping."

I wasn't. I was just sitting in my room, lights off, door closed.

I've come to understand that isolation is a symptom, not a solution. It feels like safety, but it's a trap. It keeps you from being seen, sure, but it also keeps you from being helped. And silence wasn't peace. It was punishment.

In isolation, I perfected the disappearing act. Not dramatic, not walking out the door, not vanishing into a bottle. It was quieter than that. I'd be right there in the room but already gone. Sitting at the dinner table with my jaw locked. Coaching at the rink but checked out before the puck even dropped. Pretending to watch TV beside Lizzie while my mind spun in circles miles away.

It's a cruel trick, disappearing without moving an inch. My body was still there for them, but the man inside had already left. And the silence kept the door locked behind him. Sometimes, in that silence, the old hum would return. Not a loud cry, just a background frequency of despair: *I wanna die*. A reminder of the easiest way out.

And then, a new voice would speak. Calm. Clear. Coming from another part of my mind. It didn't scream. It simply observed, like a strategist assessing a map:

Now is a good time.

It would point out the open garage, the sharp tools, the quiet house. It would note the sharp curve in the road up ahead on my drive to work. It wasn't a command. It was a presentation of facts. An opportunity. And the most terrifying part was its logic. In the middle of the storm, it sounded like the only sane voice.

It was a siren song sung by my own broken nerves, and for a long time, I didn't know how to block my ears.

That's the part that almost killed me, not the grief, not the anger, not even the trauma. It was the silence. The vanishing. The way it stole me from the people who were still right there.

I'm trying to claw my way back. Still trying to show up. Even if it's just once a week. Even if it's just a cup of coffee with a friend. Even if it's just opening the door and walking outside to watch the kids play instead of sitting behind the curtain.

Some days I make it. Some days I don't. But I'm trying. That counts for something.

Because disappearing is easy. Reappearing, that's the hard part.

Chapter Eight
She Stayed

I really only started to feel the storm I was in back in 2019, before the world went sideways. I got hit with meningitis, hard. It wasn't just illness. It was an annihilation. The headaches weren't headaches; they were a white-hot ice pick driven through my temple and out the other side. The slightest light, the glow from a phone screen, felt like a sun exploding inside my skull.

I remember being hunched over in the passenger seat of my own truck, my forehead pressed against the cold glass, trying to escape the fire in my head. Rannon was driving, his hands tight on the wheel, too quiet. I could feel his fear. Every bump in the road was a fresh agony. Lizzie had to get the kids to school first. The logic of that, the sheer, brutal practicality of motherhood, echoed in the space between waves of pain. Of course. The world doesn't stop.

I remember thinking, *This is it. This is the pain that breaks you*. It wasn't a fear of death, not exactly. It was a certainty that this pain was infinite, that every inch of me was simultaneously on fire, bruised, and bleeding internally, and that it would never, ever end. It was the first time I truly felt my body was not my own but a hostile country I was trapped inside.

That knocked me on my ass for weeks. I was sick, weak, foggy. For a while, I thought I might not bounce back at all. And when I finally got upright again, something in me was different. Slower. Heavier.

They gave me oxy for the pain. I looked at the bottle and thought, *This is how it starts*. I'd seen what pills could do. I was terrified of becoming a cautionary tale, some guy who survived the military just to spiral on a prescription. So, four days in, I ditched the pills and started smoking instead. Weed wasn't about fun. It was about function. It dulled the volume, numbed the ache, helped me stand up straight when nothing else did.

I didn't call it self-medication, not then. But that's what it was. I had demons I couldn't name, and getting high kept them at bay, at least for a little while.

Then came COVID.

The world shut down and everything stopped, but the noise in my head didn't. If anything, it got louder. The isolation hit different. The routine was gone. Everything got weird. Days bled together. I lost track of time, of purpose. There was this heavy, surreal stillness in the air, and I was already running low before it started. The pandemic just pressed harder on an already full cup.

I wasn't me. Not really. But I didn't know how to say that out loud. So, I didn't.

Instead, I got angry at small things. Stupid things. A drawer that stuck. A missed email. A spilled cup of milk. I'd snap. Not explode, snap. Just enough to scare the people closest to me. Just enough to make my kids flinch and my wife go quiet. I didn't recognize it as trauma. I just thought I was failing.

So, weed became my armor. Light up, breathe deep, dull everything. I convinced myself I was still functioning, still present. But I wasn't really. I was ghosting my own life in real time.

We stopped connecting, Lizzie and I. We were roommates with shared logistics. There were nights I'd sit next to her on the couch and feel a mile away. She'd ask how I was. I'd grunt. She'd press. I'd deflect. Eventually, she stopped asking.

There was a moment, I don't even remember what sparked it, where she looked at me, and I swear to God, it was like she didn't recognize the man sitting in front of her. And honestly? I didn't either.

The unraveling wasn't loud. It wasn't a fight. It was the distance. The silence. The way we both moved around each other like furniture.

There was a one time, months after the meningitis, when my body tried to shut me down completely. I was leaving work one evening, turned onto the road, and that was the last thing I remembered. Next thing I knew, I heard OnStar talking to me, and a cop was at my window. My truck was wrecked. Airbags deployed. I was lucky I didn't hit anyone else or die right there.

I didn't know then that my body was waving a red flag. That it couldn't keep carrying everything I'd refused to feel. Looking back now, I can see it clear as day: I just didn't know how to listen.

Not too long after that came the panic attack.

I thought I was dying. Heart pounding, chest tight, couldn't swallow. My vision tunneled and my limbs went cold. It felt like I needed to be snapped in half, like a stick, just broken right down the middle to release the pressure. The feeling made no sense, but it was all consuming.

I told Lizzie to call 911. I didn't care if it was embarrassing. I thought that was it.

The EMTs checked me out. Said it was just PVCs. "Premature ventricular contractions. Nothing major." I nodded like I understood, like that made it better. But it didn't. I felt stupid. Like I'd wasted everyone's time. Like a fraud.

We didn't really tell the kids anything. What do you say? "Dad had a moment"? "Dad's falling apart"?

There was one moment, after all the migrant ops, after the funerals, after the early cracks started to show, that I'll never forget. We got a call about a whale tangled in fishing gear. Just a routine check. Nothing urgent. But when you're trying to find a singular whale in the middle of the goddamn ocean, it feels like a joke.

We launched the small boat anyway. Searched for a while. Saw nothing. Then I looked up. I looked at the sky and asked for help. I don't know who I was talking to. Jay. God. The sea.

A minute later, the whale surfaced. Not a miracle. Not proof of anything. But I felt something. Like maybe I wasn't alone. Like maybe he was still with me.

The whale lifted its fin, slow and heavy, almost like it was saying *Please help me.* That image is burned into me. We were scared. A giant whale against our small boat. Could we even get close? Could we even do anything?

The order came to stand down and wait for the NOAA whale entanglement team. They were the experts. We weren't. So, we circled, helpless, watching. And then, before the team ever arrived, the whale slipped beneath the water and was gone.

Another chance lost. Another thing I couldn't save. Just another moment in my life where it felt like something had slipped through my hands and disappeared.

It's one of those things I don't talk about often. Doesn't make sense said out loud. But I carry it.

Captain T tried to keep me in. He was the kind of guy who could talk the balls off a pool table. Half myth, half walking, swearing, tattooed, and tanned legend. Salty as hell, but sharp. A lifer in every sense, and he saw something in me. When things started to go sideways and I was debating getting out, he did what he could. Pulled strings. Made a few calls. Offered me a tour in Newport. Shore duty. Something easier. Something stable.

And I thought about it. I really did.

There is a version of my life where I took that billet. Where I wore the uniform a few more years, collected a few more ribbons, tucked a few more memories into the box. But every time I tried to picture it, I couldn't breathe. The idea of staying in, of staying gone, of giving more of myself to something that had already taken so much—I just couldn't do it.

"I need to be home," I told him.

It felt like quitting. Like letting him down. But it was the only truth I had left. I was already fading, and if I didn't go then, I wasn't sure I'd ever get myself back.

Years later, I still wonder what would've happened if I'd said yes. If I'd stayed in. If I'd taken Newport. But I didn't. I came home. And maybe that's really where the next storm began.

There was a time Lizzie and I weren't talking, not really. Just circling each other in a house heavy with everything unsaid. And then Mother's Day came.

Lizzie told me she needed a break. Just a night to herself. She got a hotel room right in town. Nothing dramatic. No big scene. She just . . . left.

She didn't ask me to go with her.

And I don't think I would've said yes if she had, but still, she didn't ask. And that wrecked me. It felt like a quiet verdict on how far I'd drifted.

Later she told me she dropped her bag in the hotel room, just a gym duffel with yoga pants, a toothbrush, and her book club's latest romance novel. She ran the shower scalding hot until her skin turned pink. She let herself cry for the first time in weeks, the kind of crying that comes from so deep you forget it's there until it breaks open.

Her phone buzzed.

Declan: "Did u take my blue Gatorade?
Mairin: " Can I use ur lip gloss?

Nothing from me.

She went downstairs, sat at the hotel bar, and ordered a drink. She said it felt like a small rebellion, sitting alone, anonymous, surrounded by strangers who didn't know or care what she was carrying.

She watched the restaurant side, busy with normal families. Normal chaos. She watched a dad weave a stroller around. Saw him laugh when the baby spit up on his shirt.

We used to laugh.

When did we stop?

Was it after Jay died? After Flynn was born screaming? After the third night she'd found me passed out in the garage, reeking of weed and despair?

She knew the script:

He's trying.

He's hurting.

He'll come back.

But what if he didn't?

What if the man she married was buried under so much armor, he'd forgotten how to take it off?

She almost called. Almost.

Then she pictured my face, that vacant stare, jaw tight, eyes miles away, and dropped the phone.

Let him wonder.

Let him hurt.

Let him miss me.

She finished her drink and went upstairs. She said she slept like the dead.

Meanwhile, back at home I was spiraling. Big time. My mind took every exit ramp to worst case scenario land. *She left. She's not coming back. This is it.*

I didn't sleep. I paced. I smoked. I stared at the walls and built entire conversations in my head that never happened. By the time she came home, I was a shell. Angry. Hurt. Resentful.

And then, like always, she just walked back in. Calm. Collected. Recharged.

But I couldn't let it go. I told her everything. All the stories I'd built while she was gone. All the twisted truths I'd convinced myself of. I didn't yell. I didn't accuse. I just unloaded.

That's when I knew I wasn't inviting her in. I was pushing her out. My fear had become a weapon, and I was swinging it at the one person still standing beside me. I was treating love like a threat and wondering why I felt alone.

That night was a turning point. That's when I knew we needed help. That's when I knew I needed to let her in.

And when I did, I realized that through every shutdown, every moment I wasn't the man who she married, Lizzie stayed.

She stayed when I pulled away. Stayed when I shut down. Stayed when I lashed out at the world and numbed myself to everything else.

She protected the kids from the worst parts of me. Kept the house running. Showed up even when I didn't.

She didn't yell. She didn't give ultimatums.

She just . . . stayed.

It was after that I agreed to therapy. Not the bullshit kind. Real help. I was out of tricks.

And now that I was finally ready to start fixing what I'd broken, she didn't say, "I told you so."

She said, "Okay. Let's go."

And we did. We went to couple's therapy. That was the start of finding my way out of the storm.

Those sessions were uncomfortable, raw, sometimes even brutal, but they were also times I stopped pretending and started letting Lizzie in. And it didn't take long before the counselor and Lizzie and everyone in the room was saying the same thing: "You need to do this for yourself too."

That was when I first stepped onto the road to healing. Not sprinting, not even walking steady. Just a step. But it was enough to keep me from drowning.

I don't know what kind of strength that takes. But I know I wouldn't have made it without it.

Chapter Nine

DIAGNOSIS

It took at least a few days for it to sink in, but the shame came hot and fast. What would the guys at the yard think if they knew? Would they see a victim? A liability? A guy who couldn't handle his shit? I'd built my identity on being the one who could fix things, who had the answers. This diagnosis felt like a verdict: Permanently Broken. Unfixable.

I felt like an imposter. I hadn't seen combat. I hadn't watched a buddy die in my arms on some foreign soil. My trauma was quieter, a slow leak, a series of losses and moral injuries that had pooled inside me until I was drowning in it. Who was I to claim this title? Did I even deserve it?

I'd survived. Jay hadn't. DC hadn't. And here I was, getting a medal for my own breakdown.

The guilt was a familiar coat I put on. It still fit. The diagnosis didn't feel like an answer; it felt like a confirmation of a failure I'd always suspected was there.

Later, I read it off a sheet of paper like it was someone else's story. Didn't cry. Didn't panic. Just stared at it, blinked a few times, and went back to work. I had the folder in one hand and a pen in the other. I was supposed to be reviewing parts inventory, but I couldn't read the numbers. They floated. Disconnected.

I sat at my desk for a while with my jaw locked. That muscle in the side of my face, the one that always tensed up during stress, was twitching. I stared at the corner of the computer monitor until my eyes watered. Then I stood up, walked outside, and leaned on the edge of the railing, Just breathing. Salt in the air. Fiberglass dust. Diesel smoke. Normal things. But I wasn't normal anymore.

The word sat in the back of my throat like gravel. Heavy. Familiar. I'd known it was coming, long before someone said it out loud.

I didn't feel like I deserved it. I wasn't a war hero. I was just broken. Tired. Angry. Numb. Jumping at sounds that didn't bother anyone else. Losing track of time. Forgetting simple things. Avoiding the people I loved. Hating myself more than I'd ever admit.

And then there was the guilt and shame. Like I was stealing valor just by being diagnosed.

But the more I sat with it, the more it made sense. It explained everything I'd never had the words for.

Her office smelled like lavender and printer paper. There was a sound machine humming in the corner, pink accented everything, and those little plastic plants on the windowsill trying to make the place feel soft. It didn't. It felt like a waiting room with a couch. She was running late that day. Funny enough, I wasn't even mad about it. Gave me more time to brace.

When she finally walked in, she was wearing one of those Lilly Pulitzer dresses she always wore, bright, floral, like she refused to let the weight of the job stain her. Clipboard in hand. Calm. She didn't ease into it. Just sat down, crossed her legs, and said it.

"Well, you scored high on the assessment. You have PTSD."

Just like that. Like she was reading off a lab result. Like she'd just told me I had strep throat and here's your prescription. But it wasn't strep. It was a diagnosis that rewired everything I thought I knew about myself.

I nodded. Maybe blinked. I heard the words, but they didn't land right away. They floated. Disconnected. I smiled a little. The kind of smile you give when you don't know what else to do. My ears were ringing and my chest went tight, but I didn't say a word.

I don't remember much of what came after. I think she talked some more. I think she handed me a printout. I nodded again. I remember walking back to my truck, sitting in the driver's seat, and staring at the steering wheel like it might give me instructions.

Everything felt slow and loud at the same time. I wasn't angry. I wasn't sad. I was . . . hollow. Not surprised, just emptied. Like someone had finally given language to the thing I'd been dragging behind me for years, and now that it had a name, I wasn't sure I wanted it.

The worst part wasn't the diagnosis. It was how easily I slipped back into pretending nothing had changed. I still folded laundry. Still answered texts. Still showed up to work. I'd hand off repair orders and check fuel logs while this invisible storm raged just behind my eyes.

The guys at the yard didn't know. How could they? I still smiled, still cursed at broken bolts, still played the part. But underneath, everything was cracked. There were days I had to walk into the head just to be alone. Not to cry. I couldn't even get there emotionally. Just to breathe. To stop shaking. To count tiles or stare at the floor until my hands stopped clenching.

PTSD.

Letters that felt borrowed. Like I'd stolen someone else's war.

On a whim, I asked Lizzie for a date night. We decided to get tattoos. I sat in the car, engine off, staring at the tattoo parlor. Neon sign glowing "Cape Cod Inked." The kind of thing Jay would've laughed at.

No plan. No sober thought. Just an itch under my skin, the kind that used to drive me to liquor stores or barstools. Now it drove me here.

A bell jangled when we walked in. An artist with purple hair and covered in tattoos looked up from her phone. "Can I help you?" Told her I was looking to get knuckle tattoos. "What's the word?"

I didn't hesitate.

"Hold fast."

She nodded. Like she'd heard it before. Maybe from other broken men.

The chair smelled like lavender and alcohol. She wiped my hands. Cold. Sharp.

"You're gonna feel this," she said.

Yeah, I already do.

The needle bit. Black ink pooling. Skin stinging.

H-O-L-D. Right hand. F-A-S-T. Left.

I thought about Jay's grip on his chest, tendons taut like rigging. I thought about Lizzie silently lacing her fingers with mine in the ER. I thought about the migrant kid's hand clutching that gasoline-soaked shirt.

Blood beaded. The tattoo artist wiped it away. Kept going. "Navy?" she asked.

"Nah. Coast Guard."

"Figured. You guys love this shit."

I flexed my fists. Letters still raw but mine. Back in the car. Hands on the wheel. White knuckled. Words staring back at me. Lizzie rolled her eyes. "Dramatic." The kids would ask to touch it. The guys at work wouldn't mention it.

Later that night, I stood at the bathroom mirror. Toothpaste foaming. Knuckles throbbing. The man in the glass looked tired. Older. Like he'd been fighting something he couldn't name.

Now he had the name. And a reminder.

HOLD FAST

Hold fast.
Not a plea.
A command.

Another night not long after the diagnosis, we went to Mairin's dance recital. Her big night. And God, I could watch her dance forever. That girl radiates joy. No nerves, no fear, just movement and light. It was the kind of night that should've felt easy. Beautiful even. But I was fraying under the surface.

Flynn completely lost it midshow, screamed during a quiet moment, flailed in his seat. I remember gripping the chair like it might anchor me. I was doing everything I could to keep it from falling apart—him, me, the moment. But Mairin never flinched. She just kept dancing. That's who she is.

And for a second, I wasn't drowning. I was just a dad in the dark, watching his daughter shine. The weight I'd been carrying, Flynn's chaos, Declan's fire, my own unraveling, flickered quiet for a moment. She didn't just dance. She reminded me there was still something worth holding onto.

And then it passed. The lights came up, the applause faded, and we shuffled out into the night like everyone else. But I carried that flicker home. I still do.

I didn't say much on the ride home. None of us did. Lizzie sat quietly beside me. She didn't ask how I was doing. I don't think she needed to. I had that look, the one she'd seen before. The one I thought I hid. Maybe she was tired too. Maybe she didn't want to poke the bear. Maybe she just knew that silence was the only safe thing we had left that night.

I didn't tell anyone how close to the edge I was. I couldn't. I was afraid of what they'd say or, worse, what they wouldn't. I had this fear that if I said it out loud, everything would unravel. That I'd lose my job. That I'd be seen as unfit. That someone would take my kids away.

So, I smiled. I made small talk. I joked with parents in the parking lot. But inside, I was barely holding on.

People talk about putting on a brave face like it's a choice. Some days it didn't feel like I had one. It was just the mask I'd worn so long, it fused to my skin.

Silence was always the real enemy.

On the cutter, it was the silence after the engines cut and all you could hear was your own breathing. At Jay's funeral, it was the silence between my words, the kind that made my suit feel like a coffin. At home, it was the silence after doors slammed, and Mairin hid in her room.

Silence is how I learned to disappear, even in a full house. It was my isolation, my punishment, my shield. It almost killed me.

So I broke it. Not clean, not all at once. First with Lizzie when I told her the stories I'd built in my head while she was gone, then in therapy work. Then with my kids, when I let them see the cracks instead of pretending I was fine. And finally, here on these pages, where silence doesn't win because I won't let it.

My body is a ledger of what I couldn't say out loud. A skeleton with bagpipes for DC. Swallows for Jay. Dog tags for my father. A lion for the fight. Anchors for the sea. The names of my children, written where I can never forget them.

And across my hands, *Hold Fast.* Not just ink. Not just tradition. A promise.

Not everything was saved. Not everyone made it home.

But I did, and now I know that the silence doesn't get the last word.

Chapter Ten
After the Storm

I used to think getting a diagnosis would fix everything. That putting a name on what was tearing me apart would somehow make it less sharp. Less dangerous.

It didn't. Not exactly.

But it did give me a map.

For years, I kept moving like nothing was wrong. Working. Coaching. Parenting. Smiling for photos. All the while carrying this silent war inside me, convinced I had to fight it alone.

Now, I know what I'm fighting—post-traumatic stress disorder. Words that felt foreign at first. Like they belonged to someone else. Like they were not mine.

But the storm was there all along, and giving it a name didn't cure it, but naming it helped me learn to navigate through it.

Therapy helps.

I won't pretend it's magic. It's not a neat arc where you start broken and walk out fixed. Some days, I leave therapy feeling heavier than when I went in, like we dredged up the sludge from the bottom of the harbor, and now it's floating around, clouding the water.

The day after therapy is almost always the hardest. I call it the hangover. My brain feels bruised, my chest tight. Sometimes I snap at the kids over nothing or drift off in the middle of conversations. It's like we stirred up ghosts, and they follow me around, whispering old stories. But the truth is, it has to come up before it can go out.

Sharon, my therapist, is calm but sharp. She listens without flinching, even when my stories get dark. She asks questions that hit like sledgehammers:

"What do you think you lost that day?"

"What would it mean if you let yourself be angry at him?"

"When did you first learn to disappear?"

Sometimes I answer. Sometimes I just stare at my hands, counting the freckles on my knuckles to keep from crying.

She has this way of sitting in silence that makes me feel seen instead of judged. When I start circling, talking too fast, skipping details, trying to outrun the story, she doesn't interrupt. She just waits. Let's me burn myself out. Then she drops one of those questions that cuts right through. Sometimes it catches me off guard. Sometimes it breaks me open. But it always lands.

We talk a lot about triggers. But we also talk about the quietest thoughts. The ones I'd never given voice to. I had to confess to her, and in doing so, to myself, that for months my greatest nightly wish was to not wake up. That I'd hummed my own death wish like a lullaby because the noise in my head was too loud for anything else. That I'd felt overwhelming, shameful disappointment each morning when I found I'd survived another night.

Admitting that was like admitting I'd been trying to quietly evaporate from my own life. She didn't flinch. She just nodded and said, "That is a profound level of pain; thank you for telling me." And for the first time, I felt the weight of that pain lessen, because I wasn't carrying it alone anymore.

She gave me a grounding technique: Five things I see, four I feel, three I hear, two I smell, one I taste. I thought it was bullshit at first. But the other night, I was standing in the kitchen, heart racing, fists clenched, and I tried it.

I see the blue coffee mug.

I see the chipped tile on the floor.

I see Mairin's drawing on the fridge.

I see the dog's food bowl.

I see Lizzie's hair tie on the counter.

By the time I got to taste, I could breathe again.

It's not a cure, but it's a tool. And that's something I didn't have before.

I'm learning that healing isn't about going back to who I used to be. That version of me is gone. And maybe that's okay.

Because the man I've become knows things that earlier version of me didn't.

I know how to breathe through a panic attack instead of spiraling into fear.

I know when to step outside so my kids don't catch the edge of my storms.

I know how to say, "I'm not okay," without shame.

I know I'm not the only one feeling this way.

Life now is quieter in some ways, but also deeper.

Mornings start early, like they always have. Coffee. A couple stretches to unlock the knots in my back. The dog usually finds me before anyone else does, tail thumping the cabinets.

I'm still not a fan of quiet rooms. I keep music on in the background, just enough to keep the silence from closing in. Lately, it's been Phish, some old Grateful Dead tracks, or even the country music that Lizzie and Declan like.

Work is steady. Same marina, same diesel engines humming, same smell of salt and fiberglass. I still carry a notebook and bark orders when I have to. But I'm different now. I'm softer around the edges. More willing to admit when I'm tired or when something's eating at me.

Sometimes, I'll be halfway through a job and just . . . pause. Stand at the end of the dock, watching sunlight glitter across the water, thinking how for years I never let myself be still like this.

My marriage carries the dents and scars inflicted during those earlier years. There's no denying that.

But Lizzie's still here. Still beside me.

Some nights, we talk for hours. Other nights, we sit on the couch in silence, just letting the weight settle without trying to fix it. She's learned to read my signals. She knows when to give me space and when to pull me back.

I used to think love was all grand gestures. Big speeches. Dramatic vows. But Lizzie taught me it's quieter than that.

Like bringing home toilet paper when the house is out, because she knows the last thing I want to do is go into a crowded store.

Like pausing midsentence when she sees my jaw tighten.

Like sitting beside me when I'm silent, not asking me to talk until I'm ready.

Sometimes I look at her and wonder how she didn't leave. How she managed to hold our family together when I kept disappearing inside myself.

She's the reason I kept trying.

There was a night not long ago when we were in the kitchen after the kids went to bed. The dishes were piled up; the dog was snoring under the table. Lizzie turned to me and said, "You laugh more these days."

It hit me like a punch. Because I hadn't noticed.

I wanted to say thank you. I wanted to tell her how many nights she saved me without even knowing it. But instead, I just pulled her in and rested my forehead against hers.

Some things don't need words.

The kids are getting older now.

Rannon's a man. Sometimes I look at him and forget for a second that he was ever the kid in the car seat, riding around Cape Cod with me blasting music. He's steady. Quiet. But I see flashes of me in his humor, in the way he stands when he's trying to act like nothing bothers him.

Declan's still fire on the ice. He's playing high school hockey now, and every time he steps into the rink, I hold my breath a little. Not because I'm worried about his skills but because I'm worried about how much of me he's carrying. The pressure. The rage. The need to prove something. I'm trying so damn hard not to let my storms become his.

There was a game not long ago where Declan took a rough hit and went down hard. My chest locked up. I wanted to climb over the boards and fight the kid who did it. But I stayed put. Lizzie caught my eye and gave me the smallest nod. A reminder that Declan needs a dad, not a brawler.

After the game, Declan came out of the locker room smiling., no worse for wear. And I realized I was the only one still carrying it.

Mairin is still my soul guide. She's older, smarter, even more perceptive. The other night, I came home tired, face tight, shoulders hunched. She looked up at me and said, "It's a heavy day, huh, Dada?"

I nodded. She just hugged me. No fixing. No questions. Eight years old, teaching me how to be human.

She made me a bracelet recently. Plastic beads spelling out "Hold Fast." I wear it sometimes under my jacket sleeve. She doesn't know how perfect that phrase is for me.

Flynn's a tornado. Three years old and unstoppable. He's pure joy—sticky fingers, big belly laughs, and the kind of curiosity that makes me believe the world might still be a good place. He doesn't know my history. He doesn't care. He just wants me to chase him around the living room. Sometimes I do.

I still have bad days. Days when I feel the hum under my skin. Days when I leave work exhausted from holding myself together. Days when I stare out the window and wonder how the hell I'm still here.

There are days when the memories come crashing back uninvited—the phone call about Jay, the migrant boat, the silence in Rockland, the look in Lizzie's eyes after one of my outbursts.

But there are good days too. Days when I laugh without forcing it. Days when I stand in the rink and actually see the game instead of drifting somewhere else. Days when Mairin climbs into my lap, and I stay present instead of pulling away.

The rink feels different these days. I'm not behind the bench anymore. No whistle, no clipboard, no pacing like the whole game depended on me. I just walk the rails with a coffee, leaning on the glass, watching.

The sounds hit the same—skates carving, pucks off the boards, the Zamboni growling in the corner. The smell too, that mix of sweat and cold air that never really leaves your jacket. But my chest doesn't lock up like it used to. I'm not wound so tight.

Sometimes I talk with the other parents. Sometimes I don't. Declan doesn't look up in the stands as much, and that used to sting. Now I think maybe it's because he doesn't need to check if I'm about to snap. He knows I'm there. He knows I'm steady, even if I'm just standing there with my coffee.

I miss coaching, sure. I miss being part of the bench. But I don't miss the pressure I put on those kids or the pressure I carried myself. Walking the rink now, I can finally just let the game belong to them.

Sometimes, late at night, I go out to the garage and put on a song Jay loved, usually U2 or the Beastie Boys. I close my eyes and listen.

And for a moment, it's all there: the Coast Guard ships, the hockey benches, the hospital hallways, the funeral lilies, the kids' laughter, the weight of silence, the hum of healing.

All of it.

I breathe it in. I let it hurt. I let it remind me that I'm still alive.

I'm still standing.

Still holding fast.

Chapter Eleven
The Unsent Letters

Dear Boys,

I didn't write this before now because I couldn't explain myself. I left so much unsaid, hoping the weight would lift on its own. But life doesn't work that way. And you all deserve more from me than silence.

First, know this: Nothing you ever did brought me pain. Quite the opposite. You were my reason to stand up when I wanted to disappear. You made me laugh when I thought I couldn't anymore. You made me proud in ways no uniform, no ribbon, no title ever could.

If you ever saw me struggling and didn't understand why, if I seemed far away or heavy, it wasn't you. I was often at war with ghosts. Some old. Some that looked like people I loved. Some that lived only in my head. And some I wore like armor so no one could see I was scared.

There were times I didn't know how to show you the kind of father I wanted to be. I was tired. I was lost. I left part of myself out there on the water, in the uniform, in the silence that followed. But I never, not for a second, stopped loving you. And I never stopped hoping you'd grow up to feel safe, strong, and seen—even when I didn't know how to model that.

Whatever you become in this life, whatever dreams you have, whatever detours or mistakes you make, know that you can always come home. You can always call me. You can always be exactly who you are.

No masks. No pretending. Just you. And me. And the love that never left.

I'm proud of you. Not for what you do. But for who you are.

Love,

Dad

Unsent Letter to Mairin

My Sweet Girl,

There's probably a lot you've felt that I never put words to. And maybe you won't remember all of it, but I do.

I remember the times I came home carrying stuff I should've left at the door. Storm in my chest. Short fuse. I'd get quiet, and you'd disappear into the toy room like that was your job. Like you already knew, stay out of the way, ride it out.

You shouldn't have had to do that. That's on me.

There were days I couldn't even look you in the eye, not because of anything you did but because I hated the version of me you were seeing. The tired one. The angry one. The one who forgot how to play.

You never called me out. You just gave me grace I didn't earn. Crawled into my lap like nothing was broken. Giggled at dumb jokes I barely had the energy to tell. You didn't need me to be perfect. You just needed me to show up. And even that was hard sometimes.

You're the only girl in this house. And something about that makes me feel like I owe you even more. Not protection, you've got plenty of your own fire, but clarity. Stability. A dad who doesn't disappear when things get heavy.

I don't always get it right. I know that. But I see you. I watch the way you carry yourself, loud and kind and fearless. And it guts me how much I want to be better for you.

I'm trying, sweetheart. Every damn day. You saved parts of me you'll never know.

Love you always,

Dad

Unsent Letter to Lizzie

Dear Lizzie,

There's so much I should've said. And so much I didn't know how to say.

You stood beside me through storms I didn't even recognize I was in. You held our family together while I unraveled, piece by piece. I know I shut you out. I know I left you alone in rooms we were supposed to share. Not just physically but emotionally, spiritually.

You deserved more. More truth. More presence. More peace.

I want you to know it was never about not loving you. It was about not knowing how to let myself be loved. I was drowning in things I didn't have names for. And you kept swimming toward me anyway.

You could've walked. You didn't.

You stayed.

And that matters more than I've ever told you.

I'm still learning how to come back to myself, to us. But I promise, I'm trying. And I see you. Everything you carried. Everything you gave.

You saved me more times than I can count.

Love always,

P

Reflections

I never gave them these letters. Maybe I never will. But writing them forced me to reckon with the man I've been. The one they've seen and the one I've hidden.

There's a quiet ache in fatherhood when you realize your kids are watching you, not for what you say but for how you carry your pain. I carried mine like a sailor, buried, locked up, silent. I thought I was shielding them. I was really just disappearing.

PTSD isn't always rage or chaos. Sometimes it's just absence. Numbness. An empty chair in the middle of the day, a father physically there but emotionally two continents away.

These letters are my bridge back.

To say I saw you. I still see you.

To remind myself it's never too late to be softer. To be known.

To remember that breaking cycles doesn't mean having it all figured out; it just means showing up anyway.

I want them to know who I am. Not the polished version. Not the broken one either. Just the real one.

Because if they can learn to be real from me, despite me, then maybe that's the legacy I leave.

I hope you win the war no one else can see.
And if you or someone you love ever feels like the weight is too much,
call or text 988. The Suicide & Crisis Lifeline is there, 24/7.

www.ingramcontent.com/pod-product-compliance
Lightning Source LLC
Chambersburg PA
CBHW020550030426
42337CB00013B/1028